What to Expect for First-Time Moms

The Ultimate Beginners Guide While Expecting, Everything You Need to Know for a Healthy Pregnancy, Labor, Childbirth, and Newborn - A New Mom's Survival Handbook

Heidi Oster

Contents

WHAT TO
Expect
FOR
First-Time Moms

A NEW MOM'S SURVIVAL HANDBOOK

The Ultimate Beginners While Expecting. Everything You Need to Know for a Healthy Pregnancy, Labor, Childbirth, and Newborn

HEIDI OSTER

Introduction

The following chapters will discuss everything that you need to know to get prepared for your pregnancy. Pregnancy is a great time, one full of excitement, and maybe a little bit of anxiety as you aren't sure what to expect. This guidebook will provide you with all the information that you need to be prepared for every step of your pregnancy.

Inside this guidebook, we are going to explore all the different parts of your pregnancy and how to be prepared. We will talk about how to pick out your OB-GYN, how to eat the right foods, what to expect during each of the different stages of the pregnancy, how to prepare for labor, and so much more!

As a first-time mother, you may be uncertain about what to expect during the pregnancy. Make sure to check out this guidebook and learn how exciting and amazing your pregnancy can be.

Heidi Oster

Chapter 1:
Pregnancy Overview

Congratulations! You're pregnant! After you have taken some time to celebrate and show off your excitement, you may be wondering what needs to be done next. As a first-time mom, you may feel overwhelmed with all the things that are on your to-do list. Some of the most important things that you need to do as you wait to meet your baby include:

Calculate the due date: You can bring out your calendar and try to figure it out, but one of the easiest ways to do it is to find a due date calculator online. It is going to tell you the date your baby is due, it can give you a calendar that shows when you can hear the heartbeat, when you find out the sex, and more.

Choose your doctor: You are going to spend a lot of time with your doctor during this time, so it is important that you find someone you see as a good match. Once you find someone, make sure you schedule your first appointment. This appointment will usually happen between six to eight weeks along.

Decide when you want to announce your pregnancy: This is different for everyone. Some will choose to tell people right away, and others may worry about the risk of a miscarriage and will wait until the first trimester is done. Some will tell family and friends but will wait to tell their boss or co-workers, because they don't want different treatment at work. You can pick the time when you tell others and even the method that you want to use.

As soon as you find out that you are pregnant, it is time to start taking care of your body. This means that you need to pay attention to your health and the foods you are eating now. You should be prepared for some of the early symptoms of pregnancy, though these are different in each person. And be aware of some of the different changes that are going to occur in your body during this time.

The important thing here is that every woman is going to be different. Just because someone else had horrible morning sickness doesn't mean that you will. And just because you are experiencing different symptoms compared to someone else doesn't mean that something is wrong. If you are ever concerned about your pregnancy, make sure to talk it over with your doctor.

Chapter 2:
Do's and Don'ts

Being pregnant can be a wonderful time. You are excitedly waiting for your new addition to come, counting down the days, wondering what they will be like and who they will grow up to be, and trying to get everything prepared. With all the new information that is coming your way, you may be confused about some of the things to expect during this new time. Let's take a look at some of the things that you should do, and some things that you should avoid, during your pregnancy.

Do Take Your Multivitamin

As we will talk about in a later chapter, eating a diet that is balanced and has plenty of healthy vitamins and minerals can be one of the best ways to provide your body with all of the healthy nutrients that you and the growing baby will need. However, your body is going through a lot right now. With that and the morning sickness that could make eating properly almost impossible, a healthy diet may not be enough.

This is why it's recommended that you take a prenatal vitamin each day. You can choose to go with a regular multivitamin, but the prenatal is often going to contain higher levels of specific nutrients that you really need when you are pregnant. Nutrients like iron, calcium, and folic acid are found in higher concentrations than regular vitamins, and they are going to help with the proper development of the fetus and can help prevent against birth defects.

Don't Smoke

Your OB-GYN should discuss this with you right away, but it is so important that you don't smoke while you are pregnant. If you are a smoker, make sure that you stop right away. Stay away from others who smoke as well.

Babies who are born to women who smoke during pregnancy are more likely to have learning disabilities and are more likely to be born at a lower weight compared to children who had mothers who didn't smoke at all. In addition, children who were born of women who smoke are more likely to experiment with smoking at a younger age and get hooked.

Try to Get Plenty of Sleep

While you are pregnant, you are likely to feel tired, like all of the time. Anxiety about the pregnancy, anticipation, and changing hormone levels can make sleep hard to come by during your nine months. Pregnancy can be really demanding, no matter which trimester you are in, and it is important for you to get the sleep that you need.

It is so important to get as much sleep as you can during the pregnancy. This means take a short nap any time that you feel tired and set a bedtime that you can stick with. Most pregnant women need to get somewhere between seven and nine hours of sleep each night. Don't feel bad if you are tired and worn down during this time. Your body is building a whole new life, and that can be exhausting. Take it easy and relax when you can.

Avid the Alcohol

Just like with the smoking that we talked about before, you also need to make sure that you avoid drinking any alcohol while you are pregnant. Alcohol can really impact the development of your baby. Women who drink any alcohol while pregnant could deliver a baby who is dealing with fetal alcohol syndrome. Symptoms of FAS could include:

- Low birth weight in the baby

- Behavior problems

- Learning disabilities

- Lagging patterns for the baby in their growth and when they hit development milestones.

The amount of alcohol does not seem to be the issue. Even smaller amounts of alcohol on occasion can still cause problems. If you run into issues with drinking during the pregnancy, it is important to talk to your doctor right away to help keep your baby healthy.

Do Add in Some Physical Activity

Sure, you may be tired and it may seem like a crazy idea to try and work out, but it is actually really good for you and for the baby. We are no longer focusing on the days when a pregnant woman needed to just sit at home and not lift a finger when they were pregnant. Exercise is good for both the mother and the baby. In addition, regular exercise during the pregnancy could help to combat many issues that come up including:

- Excessive weight gain

- Muscle pain

- Insomnia

- Mood problems

If you were someone who spent time exercising on a regular basis before you became pregnant, then it is usually fine to keep with that amount as well. You can always talk with your doctor about any of the adjustments that you may need to make to your routine. This may become more of a problem during the second and the third trimester, depending on how your pregnancy goes.

If you did not have a regular exercise routine before the pregnancy, then you should talk with your doctor about the best way to incorporate a fitness routine into your day. You will want to start out easy so that you don't cause harm to yourself or to the baby, but there is no reason that you can't start reaping the benefits of a good workout program.

Do Not Eat Any Raw Meat
Raw or any undercooked meat, as well as eggs, can carry some risk of food-borne illness. Food poisoning can also be an issue here. These conditions are hard enough on you, but they could lead to life-threatening illnesses for the baby and in some cases, if they are severe enough, could cause birth defects or a miscarriage. Make sure that all the meat and eggs that you consume while pregnant are always well cooked and prepared properly.

Eat Some Seafood
Another thing that you should consider doing when you are pregnant is to eat plenty of seafood. This seafood can be loaded with plenty of great minerals

and vitamins including iron, zinc, and omega-3 fatty acids. All of these are important for baby and for mom. Make sure that when you do eat seafood though, that it is cooked all the way through.

One thing to note here is that you should make sure that you are avoiding any fish that is raw or fish that contains higher levels of mercury because these can be harmful to the baby. Some fish that do have this higher level of mercury and should be avoided includes:

- King mackerel

- Tilefish

- Swordfish

- Shark

Avoid the Deli Meats

Deli meats may be convenient and may be something that you would like to eat on a regular basis because of their ease; they are really something that you should avoid when you are pregnant. All deli meat includes cured meats, smoked salmon, sausages, and hot dogs. These can cause a variety of food-borne illnesses like toxoplasmosis and listeriosis.

If you do decide to consume these kinds of meats, make sure that you cook them through well to reduce the risk. In addition, make sure that you eat milk and cheese that are pasteurized, not raw. You can also wash all of your produce to make sure that you eliminate any harmful bacteria that are present there.

Do Not Sit Inside of a Hot Tub

Though the idea of a hot tub may seem like a great idea to relieve some of those sore muscles and any other pregnancy-related discomforts, it is not something that you should do. This means that you should avoid things like saunas, Jacuzzis, and hot tubs. Research suggests that the heat that comes from these can be harmful to the baby and there is some research that shows how using one of the above during the first trimester could double your risk of miscarriage.

Get the Flu Shot

No matter what time of year you are pregnant, it is a good idea to go out and get a flu shot. As long as you don't have any special circumstances that would make getting the flu shot a bad thing, this is perfectly healthy. Your doctor can discuss this with you. But getting the vaccine during pregnancy not only helps you, but it can also help your baby. Your baby will not be able to get the flu vaccine for their first six months of life, so getting the flu shot during the pregnancy not only helps them during the pregnancy but also afterward.

Limit the Amount of Caffeine You Consume

While you may feel that a lot of caffeine is the only way that you are going to make it through your pregnancy, you do need to be careful about how much you are taking in. Caffeine is able to travel from you through to the placenta and will increase the heart rate of the baby. There is some research out there that suggests that you can consume up to a few cups of coffee each day and be safe. But you do not want to drink nonstop coffee and the triple-shot latte while you are pregnant. Find other ways to help you stay awake during the pregnancy to ensure that you keep the baby safe.

Be Smart About Your Weight Gain

While there is a lot of talk out there that you can "eat for two" while you are pregnant, you really shouldn't take this to heart and then eat whatever you want to. Instead, you need to be a little bit strategic about what you eat and how much you eat.

While you do need to gain a little bit of weight to help support your growing baby, gaining too much weight can actually cause more harm than good to the baby. And you probably need a lot fewer calories than you think. For example, during the first trimester, you will only need to take in about 100 extra calories each day to help your baby grow, and many times, you may end up getting less depending on how hard your morning sickness is. By the third trimester, you will probably need about 300 extra calories each day.

Avoid the Litter Box

If you have a cat in the home, then you will need to be careful. It is fine for you to pet your cat all you want, as long as you wash your hands when you are done. However, you should never clean out the litter box. Feline waste actually has millions of little parasites inside. And one of them in particular, known as Toxoplasma Gondil, can be really toxic and dangerous to mothers who are pregnant and their babies.

If you contract that particular toxin, you will never know that it is there until you start to have some complications with the pregnancy. There are no signs ahead of time, and you can't do anything until it is too late. It is possible to have a stillbirth or a miscarriage from it. And babies who contract this parasite can face a lot of serious health concerns including mental disabilities and seizures to name a few of them.

Visit the Dentist

Many people are scared of going to the dentist. The American College of Obstetricians and Gynecologists recommend that a mother who is expecting go and get routine oral health, even when they are pregnant. They also recommend that you go in to get regular dental cleanings. You should make sure that your dentist knows that you are pregnant so they can make adjustments to some of the tools they are using in some cases, but otherwise, it is perfectly safe to go while you are pregnant, and in fact, it can be good for your overall health, as well as for your oral health.

Practice Some Yoga

While you do need to be careful to not start out with something insane like hot yoga or Bikram yoga, there are many types of yoga that are fine to use while you are pregnant. You should look specifically for gentle yoga or prenatal yoga so that you can get all of the benefits without having to worry about causing harm to you or the baby. If you did not spend time doing yoga before you got pregnant, you should consider looking for a class that is designed for expectant mothers. This will ensure that you are able to practice yoga in a manner that is safe and effective for your needs. Always listen to your body and see what you are able to handle without straining too much.

Do Have Sex

There are some expecting mothers who worry about having sex because they worry about what that will do to their developing baby. Sex during pregnancy is usually just fine. If you have a high-risk pregnancy or something like placenta previa, you may want to avoid sex. But for most pregnancies, it is just fine to have sex throughout. If you are worried about having sex with your partner or you have any questions about how safe intercourse is at any time during the pregnancy, then you can always talk with your doctor about your unique circumstances.

Heidi Oster

Chapter 3:
Picking an OB-GYN

One of the first things you will need to do after finding out you are pregnant is to find your OB-GYN. This is the doctor who will care for you and your baby throughout the pregnancy. But how do you know which doctor is the right one for you?

If you already see a gynecologist who can practice obstetrics as well, you can consider asking them to help take care of you during the pregnancy. You are already familiar with this doctor so there wouldn't be any changes there. Make sure that you feel comfortable with this doctor taking care of the pregnancy and that you wouldn't mind giving birth in the hospital associated with that doctor.

If your current doctor doesn't practice obstetrics, or you don't want to use your current doctor for some reason, then you can ask for a recommendation from a healthcare provider. Sometimes you can even talk to relatives or friends who recently had a baby. Childbirth educations can provide you with this information as well.

Remember that while most families in the United States choose to deliver their babies with the help of an obstetrician, there are other options you can choose. It is possible to work with a family physician, direct-entry midwives or certified nurse midwife to name a few.

What Criteria Should I Use When Choosing My Ob-Gyn?

Each woman is going to be different and you may find that some considerations are more important for you than for others. For example, if you have things that could result in a high-risk pregnancy, you may need to see a specialist and that can change the way you look for your doctor. You may need to check with your insurance provider to see who is covered in your network. Or you might rule out a doctor who goes to a hospital too far away. Some of the other factors you may want to consider when choosing an OB-GYN include:

Your Personal Health History

If you currently have any type of chronic illness, such as diabetes, heart disease, epilepsy, or high blood pressure, you may need to talk about this with your chosen doctor. You want to have someone who has had past experience caring for patients like you. And in some cases, you may need a primatologist or a maternal-fetal medicine specialist to help with the pregnancy since both of these deals with high-risk pregnancies.

The Outlook of The Doctor

It can be really uncomfortable being in a pregnancy and then finding out the doctor holds a different outlook on some important issues. Before choosing an OB-GYN, you need to find out what the attitude is for your doctor about important issues such as episiotomies, interventions like IVs, and more. During your first pregnancy, you may not be able to predict what you will need to have happened during that time, but you can talk with the doctor and get a good idea of the general approach the doctor will use when they work with you.

If you are interested in having either a doula or other support people in the delivery room with you, then you should also discuss this with your doctor. Some doctors will only allow your partner to be in the room, and you don't want to find out about this attitude when you are delivering. You can also explore if your doctor seems supportive of you having a natural childbirth (if you choose this option), and do they encourage breastfeeding?

Compatibility

Sometimes, it all comes down to how comfortable you feel with your doctor. You could have someone who is considered the best doctor around, but if you don't like how they handle some topics, or you just don't feel comfortable with them, then this is not the right doctor for you.

Pregnancy and childbirth can be very exciting, but this is also a stressful time for some first-time moms. You want to make sure that the healthcare partner you pick out is someone who makes you feel comfortable and whom you can communicate with well. Some questions that you can ask yourself about the doctor before committing include:

- How comfortable do I feel around this doctor?

- Is the doctor going to respect my wishes during this process?

- Does this doctor seem like they will be interested in me personally?

- Did I feel like the doctor took the time to explain things to me?

- Was it easy for me to ask questions to this doctor?

How Often Will I See This Doctor?

You and your OB-GYN are going to see a lot of each other over the next few months. You will see them much more than you are used to visiting any other doctor through most of your life. This is to ensure that both you and the baby are doing well during the whole pregnancy.

At some practices, you are going to see your obstetrician at all, or at least most, of your prenatal visits. You may have the option of seeing another OB or a nurse practitioner if yours is not there. It isn't a bad thing to meet the other OBs in the office if you can because it is possible one of them could deliver your baby. In some other practices, you may see a nurse practitioner for every appointment unless you end up with a complication or you have a pregnancy that is considered high-risk.

How Many Prenatal Appointments Will I Have?

If you have a healthy pregnancy with no complications, you will still have quite a few prenatal visits to check up on you and the baby. The recommended prenatal schedule for a healthy pregnancy includes:

- Between weeks 4 and 28, you will have one visit each month.

- Between weeks 28 and 36, you will have 1 prenatal visit every two weeks.

- For the last month, weeks 36 to 40, you will visit your doctor each week.

The schedule that the doctor recommends should always be followed. It is important for you and your baby to have prenatal care. There are three times more chances that a baby has low birth weight when mothers don't practice proper prenatal care. With these regular visits, the doctor is able to spot problems and treat them, giving you the healthiest pregnancy possible.

If you are considered a high-risk pregnancy, you may need to go and visit your doctor more often. This allows the doctor more time to monitor the pregnancy and make sure that it is as safe as possible. Follow the schedule that your doctor gives to you to make sure you and your baby stay as healthy as possible.

What Happens During My Prenatal Appointments?

Many of your appointments are going to go the same. Your doctor will meet with you and ask questions about how you feel emotionally and physically and whether you have any questions, worries or complaints you will like to share. Depending on how far along you are, the doctor may have some other questions they want to ask.

The prenatal visits aim is to give the information you need to keep your pregnancy healthy and check your pregnancy as well. You should go to all of these appointments, regardless of whether you are feeling fine and think that everything is going well.

During the appointment, your doctor is going to check your urine, blood pressure, and weight. They can also listen to the heartbeat of your baby, check the position of the baby, and measure your abdomen. Each pregnancy will be a bit different so there may be other exams and tests done to check how things are going. And if the doctor sees that there may be some complications, they will closely monitor that and intervene when needed.

The findings of your every checkup will be reviewed to you by the practitioner. They will give details on what will normally happen on the next few weeks and give you warning signs to watch out for. You can also spend some time talking about the benefits and negatives of some optional tests you will want to consider.

Risk Factors That May Require Me to Visit My OB-GYN

There are some risk factors that will require you to go and visit your doctor more often than normal during your pregnancy. This often depends on your individual health profile and if any complications arise during the pregnancy. Having any of the following risk factors can help the doctor decide how many visits you should make for you to take care of your pregnancy:

Being older than 35: Most women who give birth during their late 30s and early 40s will have healthy and strong babies. However, there is a higher risk of birth defects for babies who were born by mothers aged 35 and above. Several complications during the pregnancy will also be higher.

Pre-existing health problems: There are many health conditions that can cause issues during your pregnancy and can make you high-risk. The doctor will want you to have more appointments with them when you have high blood pressure and diabetes. It is their job to ensure you that your conditions won't affect the health of you and your baby. Other conditions that could require more visits include obesity, anemia, lupus, and asthma.

Medical problems that arise while you are pregnant: While you are pregnant, your doctor is going to watch out for complications that can occur. These can include preeclampsia, pregnancy-related high blood pressure, and gestational diabetes.

Risks of preterm labor: If you show signs that you will go into labor earlier than normal, the doctor is going to monitor the pregnancy more closely.

Your mind can be at ease when you have regular prenatal visits with your doctor. By doing so, you ensure that you will have a healthy pregnancy all throughout and deliver a healthy baby at the end.

Questions to Ask Before Choosing Your OB-GYN

When you are looking for an OB-GYN, there are several questions you should ask to make sure you and your doctor are on the same page. The right questions can ensure that you get the right doctor and that there aren't any surprises later on. Some of the questions that you should consider asking before you choose your OB-GYN include:

- What are your beliefs and philosophies about birth?

- Does your doctor see birth as a medical process that needs to be managed continuously?

- Do they see birth as a process that is fraught with a lot of potential issues and requires preventative procedures?

- Do they see it as a natural process where nature should be allowed to do some of the work before interfering?

- How much choice do you think you should have in the decisions for this pregnancy?

You will have a much better pregnancy experience if you can help make decisions and are given some options. Women who feel that they are not involved and have no control over what is going on are going to have a less positive experience and may experience anxiety and depression. Choose a doctor who will let you be involved.

What Are Your Thoughts About Using Pain Relief During Labor?

Does the doctor assume that you will take the pain relief like everyone else already does, or are they there to support and encourage your whichever method that you choose?

- Will the doctor inform you about any of the side effects of the medication and pain control?

- Will they encourage you to take the pain relief or give recommendations against it if you are close to birthing?

What Are Your Thoughts About the Birth Plan?

It is important to put a birth plan together early on. While things may not always go as plan, it at least lets your doctor and others know your preferences. Talk to your doctor about it and see if they see any concerns that need to be addressed.

What Is Your Induction Rate?

Each doctor is going to have a different preference when it comes to induction. Some will discuss it after your estimated due date and some will wait until a week or more after the due date. And then there are some who will induce ahead of time to meet a schedule. Find out how often the doctor induces and see if they are happy to use it too much. Inductions can cause complications in your baby and should only be used if medically necessary.

What Is Your C-Section Rate?

C-sections can lead to a longer recovery period and most of them are not necessary. Many hospitals in the United States are showing rates of c-sections of up to 70 percent. Considering only about 10 percent of c-sections are actually necessary. It is possible that you may need a c-section during your pregnancy, but you don't want to go through one, and deal with the harmful recovery time afterward, just because it is faster and more convenient for the doctor.

Some other questions you may want to ask your OB-GYN during pregnancy and at your appointments include:

- What medications over the counter are fine for me to take?

- Is it normal to have any spotting and cramping and when should I call in about it?

- How much weight am I going to gain during the pregnancy? How much weight is acceptable, and how much is too much, for me? Can I exercise when I am pregnant?

- Do I need to get vaccinated? Which vaccines do I need?

- Will I see some permanent changes in my reproductive system after I give birth?

- Will I have any issues controlling my bladder after I have the baby?

Heidi Oster

Chapter 4:
Nutrition While Pregnant

Another topic we need to explore during pregnancy is the diet you follow. You are not going to spend your time trying to lose weight and restricting your calories. While some women may lose weight during the beginning of their pregnancy because of the morning sickness, striving to lose weight while pregnant can lead to harmful health effects for the mom and the developmental delays in the baby.

Dieting to lose weight while you are pregnant can be hazardous to you and the baby. This can be really bad because it often results in a restriction of important nutrients to the baby include folic acid and iron. This is why you should avoid some of the popular diet plans, such as South Beach, The Zone, Atkins, and the Raw Food Diet while you are pregnant.

When we talk about diet while pregnant, we mean fine-tuning some of your eating habits so that you and the baby get plenty of good nutrition. Healthy eating during this time is so important to the development and growth of the baby. To get the nutrients that are needed, you must eat from a variety of food groups, while also limiting your consumption of junk foods, sugars, and processed foods. Yes, you may have a lot of different cravings during pregnancy, and it is fine to give into them on occasion, but overall, you do need to limit your consumption of these.

Remember that while you are pregnant, you do not need to eat for two. Many pregnant women fall into this mindset and then find they have put on way too much weight during their pregnancy. In the beginning, you will only need about 100 extra calories a day. During the final trimester, when the baby gets big and needs more nutrition, you can have up to an extra 300 calories each day.

The Food Groups to Eat

When you are pregnant, it is important to eat a wide variety of foods through-out the day. Doing this will make sure that you yourself and your baby the nutrients you both needs. Some of the food groups that you should concen-trate on during this time include:

Fruits and Vegetables

Fresh produce contains many of the important nutrients that you need for pregnancy. They are especially high in folic acid and vitamin C. While you are pregnant, you must get in a minimum of 70 mg of vitamin C each day to help keep you healthy. You can find plenty of this nutrient in vegetables like Brus-sel Sprouts, tomatoes, and broccoli and in fruits like honeydew, grapefruits, and oranges.

To help prevent any neural tube defects in your baby, you need to take in 0.4 mg of folic acid every day. Dark leafy vegetables can help provide you with this folic acid, and legumes, like veal, black-eyed peas, and lima beans are good sources too. Try to get about two to four servings of fruit each day, and at least four servings of vegetables.

Bread and Other Grains

One of the main sources for energy when you are pregnant will be the carbs that are found in grains and breads. You need to make sure that you take in enriched products and whole grains because they provide the body with many great nutrients, including Iron, fiber, protein, and the B vitamins. You can sometimes get extra folic acid if you eat fortified cereals and bread.

The amount of grains that you should consume each day will depend on your weight as well as your personal dietary needs. You can have somewhere between six to eleven servings of these grains and bread each day.

Protein

Don't forget to get in plenty of protein into your diet during pregnancy. Beans, eggs, fish, poultry, and meat can all be great sources of protein. They also contain much of the iron and B vitamins that you need. Remember that not only do you need protein, but your growing baby needs it in higher amounts during the second and the third trimester. Iron is also important because it helps to carry oxygen to the baby. Your body needs oxygen as well because it moves oxygen to your muscles, which can help alleviate pregnancy symptoms like depression, irritability, weakness, and fatigue.

It is recommended that you take in about 27 mg of protein each day. There are a lot of great options when it comes to choosing where to get your protein from each day. Lean beef, liver, veal, turkey, lamb, and chicken can be good. Some types of fish and other seafood can be good, as long as you follow the right guidelines. Aim to consume a minimum of three servings of protein each day.

Dairy Products

During pregnancy, you should consume a minimum of 1000 mg of calcium each day. Calcium is so important to building up strong bones and teeth, to help with normal blood clotting, and can help with proper nerve and muscle function. Since your baby is going to need large amounts of calcium to help them grow and develop, your body will either need to get it out of your diet, or your body will take it from your own bones to support the baby.

There are many sources of calcium that you can choose to enjoy when you are pregnant. You can go with puddings, cream soups, yogurt, cheese, and milk. There is also a little bit of calcium found in options like dried peas, beans, seafood, and green vegetables. Make sure that you get a minimum of four servings of dairy each day.

Prenatal vitamins
Although most of your nutrition should come from the foods you eat, a daily prenatal vitamin can be useful. Sometimes, you may have trouble keeping your food down, such as during the first trimester, or you may have trouble eating as the baby gets bigger. A prenatal vitamin can help fill in some of the gaps if you need it.

Foods That You Should Avoid While Pregnant
While you are pregnant, there are also some foods that you need to avoid. These foods are often harmful because they have some bacteria or other issues with them that can harm the developing baby during this time. Some of the foods that you should make sure you avoid while you are pregnant include:

Deli meats: These types of meats can sometimes be contaminated with listeria, which can cause a miscarriage. These bacteria can cross the placenta and will affect the baby, causing infection or blood poisoning that can be life-threatening. If you do want to eat deli meats during this time, make sure to reheat them to avoid issues.

Fish with mercury: Mercury that is consumed, especially when it is done in high dosages, can be linked back to developmental delays and even brain damage. Some fish that you should use include tilefish, king mackerel, sword-fish, and shark.

Smoked seafood: Refrigerated or smoked seafood is often labeled as jerky, kippered, nova style, or lox and you should avoid it because it is likely there is listeria in it. This is the fish that is found in the deli section so avoid that.

Raw eggs: Raw eggs can have a potential of salmonella exposure, as well as foods that are made out of raw eggs, so you should avoid them. Options like Hollandaise sauces, custards, ice creams (if they are homemade), and even mayo and Caesar dressings can be an issue because they are made with raw eggs. If the recipe has been cooked at some point, this can reduce the risk.

Soft cheese: Some soft cheeses may contain listeria. You would need to avoid these such as some Mexican style cheese, Gorgonzola, feta, and brie. All soft non-imported cheeses that have been made with pasteurized milk will be safe to eat.

Milk that is unpasteurized: These types of milk can contain listeria so make sure that you drink a form that is pasteurized.

Pate: Any type of meat spread needs to be avoided because they could contain listeria.

Caffeine. While it is fine to have this in moderation, you do need to be careful with the amount. Try to keep it down to maybe one cup of coffee, or the equivalent, each day to help you not run into pregnancy complications. Drinking too much can mean that the diuretic effects of caffeine will kick in and you could end up with calcium and water loss.

Alcohol. No amount of alcohol is safe when you are pregnant and you need to avoid it the whole time. When the mother chooses to have alcohol during the pregnancy, it could interfere with the healthy development of the baby. If the alcohol is ingested in high amounts for a lot of the pregnancy, it could result in Fetal Alcohol Syndrome and other disorders for the baby. If you did drink before you found out you were pregnant, it is important to stop now. And you should discontinue your use through the pregnancy and during breastfeeding if you choose to do it.

Chapter 5:
The First Trimester Weeks 1 to 12

There is a lot that will happen with your baby as they begin to develop. The first trimester will see a lot of changes, even if you don't see your belly growing yet. You may not look like you are pregnant at this point, but it's likely that you are feeling it by now. This is because a ton of pregnancy hormones are going to work and prepping your body to host your baby for some time now. Be prepared for a lot of pains and aches from the pregnancy, and you will probably be tired quite a bit. While you might not be all that thrilled with the symptoms that come with pregnancy, remember that most of these are going to be temporary and that you get a baby at the end.

How Long Is the First Trimester?

The first week up to the thirteen weeks of your pregnancy will be your first trimester. If you are not sure when your pregnancy is, you will need to figure out your due date. This helps you to know where you are in the pregnancy and how far you have left. Remember that it is possible for the due date to change, especially if you are someone with irregular periods.

The Growth of Your Baby During the First Trimester

There is a lot of growing that your baby will go through during this first trimester. The baby will start as a zygote, a single fertilized cell. Next, it will plant itself on the wall of the uterus as an embryo where in it will continue to become a baby the size of a peach that already has limbs and body systems. Organs are going to start taking shape and the baby will start to move. Some of the other highlights that you will notice with your baby during this time include:

Their bones. When the baby reaches six weeks, they will start to grow feet, hands, legs, and arms. Their toes and fingers will start to grow at about ten weeks.

Hair and nails. Week 5 and 8 are when the baby will start forming its skin. Around week 11, the nail beds and hair follicles will form.

Digestive system. The intestines of the baby will begin to form by the 8th week. They will also have gone through two kidney sets, and the third, and final, set will be on the way.

Sense of touch. Your baby is going to start developing some touch receptors on their face, mostly on the nose and the lips, when they reach week 8. A few weeks later at week 12, they are going to have receptors at the soles of the feet, palms, and genitals.

Eyesight. By the time the baby is four weeks old, their optic nerves and lenses will start to form. By week 8, the retina will form as well.

Heart: By the time you get to week five, the tube that is going to be the heart will begin to beat spontaneously. It is going to become stronger and easier to hear sometime between week 9 and 10.

Brain. When your baby reaches week 8, their brain is going to get to work wiggling all those developing limbs.

Sense of taste. The baby is going to start developing taste buds and have them connected back to the brain by 8 weeks. But it will be some time before they can taste anything because they still need the taste pores.

Some of the other major changes that are going to occur in the baby during this first trimester include the development of their vocal cords, the production of white blood cells to help fight off any infections, and the formation of their muscles.

Changes in Your Own Body

A lot is going to happen to you during the first trimester as well. Some of the early pregnancy symptoms that you are going to notice during the first trimester include:

Morning sickness. For most women, this doesn't just strike in the morning. These symptoms are going to start up when you reach six weeks of pregnancy. There are different techniques that you can try to reduce the symptoms a little bit including taking ginger drops or tea. Stick with smaller meals. If the symptoms continue or seem to get worse, you can talk to your doctor about the options available.

Tender breasts. There will be some changes to your breasts when you are pregnant. You may notice that they get bigger, are tingly, and tender. This usually happens around week 6.

Mood swings. You may find that your mood is going to change often when you are pregnant. One moment you may be up, another time you may be down, and the next it can go all over the place. This is perfectly normal.

As the pregnancy progresses through this trimester, you may notice that there are lots of other pregnancy symptoms that come up. Each woman is different, but some of the symptoms that you may notice include headaches, food aversions, and a metallic taste in the mouth, constipation, and heartburn. The good news is that when you enter the second trimester, you should be able to get some relief from these symptoms.

Weight Gain

During this stage, your baby is still really small. This means that you are not going to gain much weight during this time. You should stick with three to four pounds of weight gain during the first trimester. If you have really bad morning sickness and can't keep food down, you may end up losing a little weight. This is fine, as long as you are able to pick up those pounds later on. For now, you should focus on eating meals that are light, but eat them more often, and make sure the foods you pick are high in nutrients. Crackers, whole grain bread, bananas, yogurt, and avocados can be great options to give you nutrients but can be gentle on the stomach as well.

For some women, they are extra hungry when they are in the first trimester. Try to keep your calorie intake in check during all parts of your pregnancy. The first trimester won't necessarily require you to have extra calories. If you do end up getting more pounds put on than is recommended during the first trimester, do not fret though. Just focus your energy on getting back on track during the rest of the pregnancy.

Symptoms You Should Have Checked Out by Your Doctor

It will be hard to know what is normal and what isn't during your pregnancy because of your body will have many different changes. In many cases, the odd twinge or a bit of pain here or there is not a big deal. However, the first trimester is going to have a higher risk of miscarriage than the others. Some of the symptoms that you should be aware of and call your doctor about will include:

- Disturbances in your vision

- Severe puffiness that shows up in the face and hands

- A fever that gest over 101.5 degrees along with chills and a backache.

- Painful urination

- A sudden thirst

- Severe abdominal pain

- Heavy vaginal bleeding.

If you do experience some of the symptoms that are listed above, it is imperative that your doctor should be notified immediately. If you are not able to talk to them right away, then you need to head to your closest ER to get help for you and the baby.

Things to Do During the First Trimester

Start your prenatal vitamin: If you haven't already started taking one ahead of the pregnancy, then now is the time to do it. The development of neural tube defect will be reduced when you take prenatal vitamins during the first trimester.

Choose your doctor: There are many different types of doctors you can choose for your pregnancy. You can work with a family physician, midwife, and OB-GYN. Take your time to look at all the options that are out there and then pick the one that best fits your needs.

Book your first appointment: You need to get this appointment done sometime between six to eight weeks. Your doctor will need to take a look at your medical history and will perform a thorough exam. You will probably go through a lot of test including a urinalysis, blood work, a Pap smear, and more. You may even get an initial ultrasound to help date the pregnancy, to check the progress of your baby, and to hear the heartbeat. While the doctor is going to ask you a lot of questions here, you should take the time to ask your own questions as well.

Consider getting some genetic testing done: There are many different types of genetic screenings that you can get done to help you be aware of what may be there with your baby. Some are noninvasive and others are more invasive. You can make a decision on whether you want to do these and which ones based on personal preferences and your family history. Taking these tests can help you be prepared for what you can expect with your baby.

Look into your health insurance: The price that you pay for your pregnancy is going to vary based on many factors such as who you visit, how many appointments you have, where you give birth, and more. You should have insurance by now or sign up for one. Look at the co-insurance and the premiums to see if you can keep your costs as low as you can.

Make a budget: When you grow your family, it is a good time to take a look at your monthly expenses and see what you can do to make sure you stay within your budget.

Eat right: Cut down on your caffeine and learn which foods you should limit as much as possible. This is an important time of growth for your baby so you need to eat foods that are high in nutrients and will keep you healthy.

Keep active: You don't have to run a marathon or anything at this point, but getting up and moving, even if it is just a nice walk outside, can do wonders when it comes to keeping you healthy, helping the baby grow, and ensuring that you feel better. It is recommended that very week; you should have physical activity for at least 30 minutes.

If you feel up to it, go ahead and have sex: Sex is allowed and just fine while pregnant, and it is safe for baby. And it can have some benefits for you as well.

Consider some baby names: While you still have plenty of time before you find out what gender you are having, this can still be a good time to start considering baby names that you will want to use.

Plan out how to announce your news: Think about when and how you would like to tell others about the news. Most women will wait until they get to the end of their first trimester to do this, but you can do it at any time that you want. You should also consider when you want to tell your boss about the pregnancy. Look up the pregnancy rules in your business to help you know what to expect.

The first trimester is an important stage of your pregnancy. The baby is developing quickly, and your body is changing as well. Make sure to schedule your first prenatal appointment early on and talk with your doctor about any concerns that you have about this pregnancy.

Heidi Oster

Chapter 6:
The Second Trimester Weeks 13 to 26

When you enter the second trimester, you are going to definitely start to see some changes in your body. The next three months are going to show a lot of changes in your baby and hopefully, the welcome relief from some of those morning sickness symptoms. For most women, the second trimester is the most comfortable one of the three. You will notice that most of your early pregnancy symptoms are going to ease up a bit, and they will disappear. You will probably not feel as queasy anymore and food may start to taste better. Your energy levels will be better and by the end, you may start to see the little bulge in your tummy that looks like the beginnings of your pregnant belly.

How the Baby Grows During the Second Trimester?

The second trimester goes from week 13 to week 26 of your pregnancy. Your baby is going to be very busy during this trimester. By the time you get to the 18th week, the baby may way as much as a chicken breast and they can do a variety of actions including hiccup and yawn. But the time you get to week 21, little jabs and kicks will be felt because of their limbs moving around. And by week 23, the baby will start to pack on the weight. In fact, for the next four weeks, the baby is going to double their weight. By the time you get to the end of the second trimester, your baby will be about two pounds. Let's look at some of the other changes that may occur to your baby during the second trimester.

Hair, nails, and skins: When you reach week 16, the initial tiny hairs of the baby will start to show up. By the 22nd week, they should have eyebrows and eye-lashes. The skin is now going to be covered in a downy fur coat, lanugo that is meant to keep them warm until they add more fat later on. And at week 21, the vernix caseosa, a greasy layer of oil that is meant to shield the skin, will show up. Both of these are going to shed off before the baby is born.

The digestive system: The digestive system of the baby will be formed fully by the time you end the first trimester. Now, the baby starts to swallow and suck in preparation to the world outside their mother's womb. They can even start to taste the foods that you are eating via your amniotic fluid. Because of this, the baby will even develop preferences based on your food choices when they are born. Choosing to eat healthy foods can help influence your baby to enjoy these same foods when they are older. In addition, the baby's waste systems are hard at work as well. The baby pees inside of the womb as well because of all that swallowing they do to get the required nutrition by the placenta.

Senses: The baby eyes and ears are working to move into the correct posi-tion, by the time the baby gets to week 22 of the pregnancy. These developing senses mean that the baby starts to hear, smell, and see, and they will start opening their eyes.

Heart: When the baby reaches 17 weeks, their heart will start beating on its own rather than spontaneously. The brain is able to control and regulate the heartbeat. Using a stethoscope by week 20, you can hear their heartbeat as well. During the 25th week, the capillaries are going to begin forming so that they are able to carry the blood around the body.

Brain: In addition to being able to control the heartbeat of your baby, and of inducing kicks, the brain is able to start getting the eyelids to blink by 26 weeks.

Changes in Your Body During This Trimester

While there are many changes that happen with your baby during this second trimester, there will also be some changes that occur in your body as well. The third trimester can bring up some symptoms from the first one, such as constipation and heartburn. As your belly keeps on growing and your hormones from pregnancy keep rising, there are some other symptoms that can show up including:

Congestion. As the blood flow starts to increase to the mucous membranes of the body, you may find that you're snoring for the first time. Some over the counter medications can be fine to use to resolve this issue.

A little swelling of the feet and ankles. This can happen in about seventy-five percent of women who are pregnant and it usually starts around the 2^{2nd} week. Some women may experience this issue a little bit earlier. To help reduce the puffiness, you should try to keep active when you can and then kick up the feet during any time you sit down. Try to avoid long periods of sitting or standing and always sleep on your side.

Sensitive gums. This can include a little bit of bleeding as well. Make sure to talk to your dentist during this time. If the gums easily bleed and are bright red in color, this might be a sign that you are dealing with gingivitis, and you need to visit your doctor.

Leg cramps. These can start during the second trimester and could last all the way to the third. This is due to both your hormones and the extra weight. And since some pregnant women may be short on magnesium and calcium, this problem could be worse. Make sure that you eat a diet that is well-balanced and healthy during your pregnancy.

Dizziness. Sometimes, pregnant women can experience low blood pressure. This is going to happen because of all that extra blood the body is trying to pump through. Make sure to drink plenty of fluids, eat plenty of small meals, and then take it easy.

Achiness in your lower stomach. This is sometimes referred to as round ligament pain. The ligaments that are supporting the belly are trying to stretch out to support the growing size of your belly.

Varicose veins or hemorrhoids. These can often shrink or even go away after pregnancy, especially if they weren't something that you dealt with before.

All of the above are considered normal during your pregnancy and they are often temporary. You may also have feelings of irritability, apprehension, frustration, and forgetfulness during this time as well.

The second trimester can bring big changes to your bedroom as well. Your sex life can be affected due to different changes that you and your partner should cope such as fatigue and nausea that can really kill the mood. However, there are some women who are going to find that they want sex more during this time. Communication is the key here to make sure that you avoid any resentment from either partner.

Weight Gain

You will start to put on more weight during the second trimester. You will start to gain weight in these next few months of your pregnancy. Your appetite is likely to increase, or it can reappear if it went away during your first trimester, to help support the growing baby. If you started out this pregnancy at a normal weight, you should gain about one pound each week, for a total of 14, during this trimester.

Symptoms You Should Check with Your Doctor On

The next few months of the second semester will relatively be a smooth ride for most women. However, there are some symptoms that can show up and if you do experience them, you should call your doctor. These include severe abdominal pain, vaginal bleeding, and a fever that is over 101.5 degrees.

This is also the time when you and your doctor will watch out for signs of gestational diabetes. This disease can start sometime between 24 and 28 weeks of the pregnancy. You may notice extreme fatigue, snoring, frequent copious urination, and extreme thirst. If you notice severe swelling, vision changes, or a sudden increase in weight, this could be a sign that you are dealing with preeclampsia.

Things to Do When You Enter the Second Trimester

The best thing that you can do during your second trimester is to make sure that you get plenty of rest, exercise regularly, and eat well. Some of the other things that you need to do during the second trimester include:

Prepare yourself for some routine monitoring: At each checkup that you do during this time, your doctor is going to do some monitoring of the baby. This includes checking the size of the uterus, checking your weight, checking out the height of your fundus, or the top of your uterus, and the baby's heartbeat. The doctor checks out all of this to ensure that the baby is growing properly and everything is going well.

Schedule your level two ultrasound: Usually, somewhere between weeks 18 and 22 of the pregnancy, the doctor is going to use an ultrasound to check on the baby. This gives them a more accurate idea of how big the baby is, how their major organs are developing properly, to determine the level of amniotic fluid, and you can even find out the gender of your baby.

Do your glucose screening: About one out of every ten pregnant women will be diagnosed with gestational diabetes. This is why the American College of Obstetricians and Gynecologists will recommend that you should be screened between 24 and 28 weeks pregnant. If the test comes back as positive for the extra glucose, it doesn't always mean that you have this disease. You will need to go through another set of testing to make sure. If you do have gestational diabetes, your doctor is going to refer you to a nutritionist who can help you create a meal plan and teach you to have to keep track of your levels of blood sugar.

Consider prenatal screening: This is a matter of personal preference. There are many women who go through their pregnancies without these tests. But if you have some risk factors or a family history, or if you just want to be prepared in case there is something, then you may want to go through a genetic testing.

Get your immunization: If you are pregnant during the winter or during the flu and cold season, make sure that you get your flu shot. Many times, it is recommended that you get the Tdap vaccine sometime during your third trimester because this helps to protect your baby against a whooping cough when they are born.

Shop for maternity clothes: Once the baby bump starts to show, you will need to get some new clothes to fit with them. Make sure to go for comfort, and get things a little bit bigger because that baby bump is just going to get bigger when you go into the third trimester.

Make sure that you sleep on your side: Sleeping on your side is the best when you are pregnant. You don't want to sleep on your stomach because this can add a lot of pressure to your baby and sleeping on your back can cause pressure on your back and your other organs.

Decide whether you want to find out the gender of the baby. During your anatomy scan, you get the option of finding out whether you are having a baby girl or boy. You can also choose to not find out at all. Consider whether you want to find out or if you want to be surprised when the baby is born.

Make your workouts a priority: Given all of the benefits that can come from a good workout program when you are pregnant, it is good to keep up with it during this time. Find a method that is good during pregnancy. Just make sure that you avoid any type of activities that aren't seen as safe for the belly, such as riding a bike or kickboxing.

Take in a few more calories: You do not need to start eating for two here, but you do need to increase how many calories you eat by a little bit to help support the baby. You will need to take in about 300 extra calories during the second trimester, which is like an extra snack or a few extra servings of product.

Track your weight gain: This is something that your doctor will help you out with by measuring when you go to your prenatal visits. At this point, you need to be steadily gaining weight. The doctor will have you keep track each week to make sure that you are staying in your limits without gaining too much.

Do some fun preparing things for your baby: Think about getting a bump shot? This is a photo shoot that shows off your baby bump before they are born. This is a good time to schedule the shot so you can get the time that you want. You can also consider taking a babymoon for your first child. Since your first-trimester nausea will be quelled, and because many airlines have restrictions on flying later in your pregnancy, the second trimester is the best option to take this trip. And you can consider what you want to add to your baby registry.

Look into some childbirth classes: While you probably won't start one of these classes until you reach the third trimester, it is a good idea to look into these classes now. This helps you to find a class that will work well for you.

Think about where you would like to give birth to your baby. Are you interested in giving birth at home, in a birthing center, or in a hospital? The answer to this question will determine a lot of things about the birth of your baby. Take some time to look into your options now. The birth centers and hospitals will often invite you to take a tour in your third trimester to help you be familiar with your surroundings, but you can do this earlier on as well.

Look into your childcare options: If you do plan to go back to your work after maternity leave is done, then it is never too early to look into some of the childcare options near you. There are many options such as a relative, babysitter, nanny, and daycare. The option you choose may depend on your personal preferences, how many hours you work, and your budget concerns.

Think about your baby shower: Traditionally, the mom to be doesn't host their own baby shower. Usually, a friend or family member will host this baby shower. But there is nothing wrong with letting your host know if you have any preferences in the theme or what is done at the baby shower. Make sure that your baby registry is done ahead of time so that well-wishers can pick out a gift.

Consider names: If you found out the gender of your baby, you will be able to narrow down the list of names that you like to correspond with the gender of your baby. There isn't a rush. You still have time to pick out a name. Some parents like exploring and narrowing down the names once they know the gender of their baby.

The second trimester is an exciting time. This is the trimester when most mothers are excited about the arrival of their baby. They have gotten through their morning sickness and some of the early morning pregnancy troubles are gone. They are able to enjoy their pregnancy and showing off their new baby bump to others. Enjoy this time. It is fun to watch your little one grow and develop like never before.

Genetic Testing

During your second trimester, you may choose to do some genetic testing. This kind of testing can be a good way to look closer at the health of your baby. Some tests are there to check the baby for a variety of medical conditions while you are still carrying them. Others are going to check the DNA to see if they carry some genetic diseases. Even before the pregnancy, it is possible for the mother and father to get a genetic carrier screening to look and see what the chances are that one of their children would get a genetic disorder.

Most of these tests are completely optional and parents can choose whether they want to get them done or not. Some parents do these in order to help them make better health decisions and to have a better idea of what they can expect when the baby arrives. Let's take a look at some of the different tests you may want to consider during the second trimester.

Triple Screen or Quad Screen

This screening is usually done sometime between fifteen and twenty weeks. These two types of multiple marker tests will check the levels of certain proteins and hormones in the bloodstream of the mother. Like other forms of screening that you may have done in the first trimester, these are noninvasive and can be done by getting the mother's blood sample.

The levels of proteins and hormones are measured from this sample of blood to help the family know how likely it is that the baby will have neural tube defects, trisomy 18, Down Syndrome, or issues with the development of the abdominal wall.

You will not have to go through a lot of preparation for this one. You just need to show up at the scheduled time to get the blood drawn. The lab and your doctor will take care of the rest.

Amniocentesis

This test is usually done sometime between fifteen and eighteen weeks, although it can be done any time that the doctor would like. It is more of a diagnostic test, which means that it can provide you with accurate information about the genetics of your baby. But it is much more invasive compared to the other options.

In addition to being able to diagnose some genetic abnormalities in your baby, this test can help you figure out other problems such as cystic fibrosis, sickle cell disease, spina bifida, and more. This test is able to detect neural tube defects about 99 percent and all genetic abnormalities 100 percent, so it is an accurate test, but invasive.

This test is done with an ultrasound. The doctor uses this to help locate the placenta and where the baby is. Then some local anesthetic is used to the area where they will insert the needle through the stomach and into your uterus. They can now remove a small amniotic fluid sample around the fetus. After this is done, you may feel a few menstrual like cramps.

Anatomy Ultrasound
This one happens sometime between eighteen to twenty-two weeks of pregnancy. This is often a standard of prenatal care that most women in the United States will use. It can help the doctor get a full look at the anatomy of the baby and is often done around twenty weeks. By this point, the major organs of the baby should be developed well and the doctor is able to see everything well.

Ultrasounds that are done earlier than the 22-week mark may need another ultrasound depending on how well the doctor is able to see everything. Usually, if the ultrasound is done at the 20th week, the doctor is able to visualize things just fine and you will only need one. This is the time where the doctor will notice if there seem to be any abnormalities and will also be able to tell the parents if they are having a boy or a girl.

CBC Blood Test

This test is done somewhere between 24 and 26 weeks. This blood test is standard and will take a look at your iron levels, thyroid function, and your vitamin D status. These are important to keep in a good range as you go through your pregnancy because they will help keep the baby strong. This procedure is done with a simple blood draw.

Glucose Screening

Your doctor will discuss this one with you as you get closer. It is usually done sometime between 24 and 28 weeks. The glucose screening, or the diabetes test as it is often called, is done in order to determine if a mother is suffering from gestational diabetes. You need to check for this during your pregnancy because leaving it uncontrolled can result in problems for you or the baby.

Women who are dealing with gestational diabetes are often likely to have large babies and can suffer a lot of problems during the delivery, including trouble with breastfeeding and dystocia, where the shoulder of the baby gets stuck. The babies can have a problem after they were born with blood sugar and may can possibly have diabetes in the future if they were born to mothers that have gestational diabetes.

A Glycol drink is used in this type of test. This drink is going to contain about 50 grams of sugar to do the test, although there are some midwives who are moving to orange juice or even jelly beans to do this test because they are a little tastier and easier on the system. With the Glycol drink, many mothers can feel sick and have a hard time with it, even if they don't suffer from gestational diabetes.

Either way, you will take the drink or the other sugary product on an empty stomach. After an hour has passed, your blood is drawn to help you determine your glucose level. Women who actually have gestational diabetes are going to have higher levels of glucose in their blood after the hour is done. If the test came out in the intermediate range, they will have to do this test again after three hours to check if they really have this issue.

To prepare, you need to go on a small fast before the screening. This ensures that none of the other foods you eat during the day will mess with the results. This is why most doctors will schedule this test right away in the morning. Have some options on hand for after the test, such as some bread or crackers, so that you can fill up your stomach when the blood test is done. Some women have had trouble with nausea and feeling sick while they take the drink, so discuss this with your doctor if you think it is going to be a concern.

If you have been able to stay on a healthy diet plan and maintain your exercise program throughout the pregnancy, then this should not be a problem for you. You can go through and do the test once and then be able to enjoy the rest of your pregnancy.

Chapter 7:
The Third Trimester Weeks 27 to 40

Welcome to the third trimester. At this point, you and your baby are about two-thirds of the way to the end. But there is still a lot of growing that your baby needs to do. It may feel at some points that there isn't a way that your belly will grow anymore. But as the baby keeps growing, your belly will grow to accommodate them as well. Here are some of the things that you can expect from the third trimester of the pregnancy.

The third trimester is going to begin during week 27 and will last until the baby is born. This can vary based on each person. Some mothers will give birth a little bit early, some will give birth right at forty weeks, and some will give birth after their due date. But the third trimester will continue going until the baby is born. In some cases, when the baby goes past the due date, you may be induced. This usually happens when you are really overdue and has reached the week 42 of your pregnancy. In the meantime, you have to get through the rest of the third trimester. The good news is that you are almost to the finish line here.

How the Baby Grows During This Time

Your baby will get bigger during the third trimester. They will grow from about two and a half pounds and sixteen inches long during the 28th week to somewhere between six to nine pound and between 19 to 22 inches long when you give birth at 40 weeks. Your baby is going to grow fast so don't be surprised when they run out of the room, and this leads to some really strong pokes and kicks in your gut.

There are a lot of things to be excited about when you reach the third trimester. Some of the highlights that you can look forward to with your baby during this time include:

The bones. As your baby starts to turn their cartilage over to bone in months seven and eight, they will start to get a lot of calcium from you. This is why it is so important during the third trimester to get plenty of foods with lots of calcium.

Hair, nails, and skin. By the time you reach the 32nd week of pregnancy, the baby's skin, which was see-through before, is going to become opaque. Then when you reach week 36, the fat will continue to accumulate on the baby, and they will have the nice plump skin that you are going to cuddle when they are born.

Digestive system. The baby's first poop, the meconium, will start to build up in the intestines in the final few weeks of the pregnancy. This waste is going to be a mix of lanugo, vernix, and blood cells.

The five senses. First, the touch receptors of the baby are going to develop when you reach week 29. By the 31st week of pregnancy, the baby is going to be able to get signals from all the senses. It can perceive the differences between dark and light, can taste what you eat, and can listen to the sounds that are around them.

Brain. During this time, the brain of the baby is going to start growing faster than ever before. They will start trying out some new skills such as regulating their own body temperature, dreaming, and even blinking.

When you get close to your 34ths week of the pregnancy, the body of the baby will turn southward so that they are settled with their head down and the bottom up. There are times when the baby won't turn around and will remain in a breech position. Around week 37, the doctor can manually turn the baby if they remain in the breech position.

Changes That Occur in Your Body

You will notice a great deal of fetal activity while the baby continues to grow and keeps busy inside you. Your body will have some changes as the baby get bigger than ever. Some of the different changes that you will notice during this time include:

Abdominal achiness. As your round ligaments, or the ones that are responsible for supporting your lower abdomen, start to stretch out to help hold onto that growing bump, it is likely that you are going to feel a sharp pain or cramps. The best thing that you can do for this is to take it easy.

Fatigue. Your body will find it hard to manage the demands of your pregnancy making you feel more tired. Try to get as much sleep as possible, stay active, and eat well to help avoid this issue.

Heartburn. In the final few weeks of pregnancy, the uterus is going to work and grow, which is going to push your stomach, as well as the contents inside, upward. This can cause a lot of heartburn for mom. If this problem is really bothering you, you may need to talk to your doctor about taking some medication to get relieved.

Braxton Hicks contractions. As the body works to prepare you for labor, you may feel a few irregular contractions. They may be a little bit uncomfortable, but they are not dangerous. They are simply a way for the body to prepare for the real thing.

Varicose veins. Some pregnant women notice that they have bulging veins in their lower body because of all the extra blood they are pumping around. The good news is that women who didn't have these before the pregnancy are unlikely to have them after the pregnancy is done.

Stretch marks. These are tiny little tears in the body because the skin is being stretched during the pregnancy. These are usually genetic, which is why some people get them really bad and others don't. Pick out a good moisturizer to help minimize the effects.

Backache. As the relaxion, a type of hormone, loosens up your joints and your growing belly pulls the center of gravity of the whole body forward, you will notice that you have an achy back. This is another reason that you should consider putting your feet up as much as possible.

Crazy dreams. Some women who are pregnant will also have crazy dreams. This is another result of crazy pregnancy hormone. Your dreams may be more vivid as you draw near the due date. This is normal.

Clumsiness. Your hormones are going to be on overdrive, you are going to be forgetful more than ever, and your belly is throwing it off balance. You are in good company. Clumsiness is something that many people deal with during the pregnancy. Just be careful and have some humor with it.

Lack of bladder control. You may want to start working on your Kegel exercises now. These will help keep you strong and can prevent a leaky bladder in the process.

Leaky breasts. Your body already knows that it will now have to feed the baby that is why it is starting to warm up. This can sometimes lead to leaky breasts if the milk comes in a bit early.

The third trimester can be hard on a first-time mom. The baby is getting big and between that extra weight from holding the baby and all the pregnancy hormones, the third trimester may feel like it is going on forever. But the finish line is almost here, and with a few more appointments and a few more weeks, you will be holding your new bundle of joy.

Symptoms That You Should Call Your Doctor About

As your due date nears, you may find that there are some symptoms of false labor that you will experience. These false signs of labor are simply your body preparing for the baby to come and they are nothing to be concerned about. However, there are a few symptoms that you need to be aware of because they are actually signs of true labor. The different signs that you should watch out for when you enter the later parts of the third trimester include:

Lightening. When you reach week 36, you may find that the baby drops down into the pelvis and you will start waddling a bit as you walk.

Blood show. This stringy mucus is going to be tined either brown or pink with some blood and it is a sign that your labor is on its way. You may or may not notice that there is a mucous plug that comes out as well. This plug is the part that seals the uterus from the outside world and when it comes out, it means that labor is coming.

Labor contractions. Compared to the Braxton Hicks contractions that some people experience, these will not diminish but rather intensify more, especially when you move.

Your water breaks. This may not happen until you are at the hospital and about to push. Each woman is different. But if you do notice that your water breaks when you are at home, you should head into the doctors right away.

Your doctor will also discuss with you the best times to call them or head into the hospital to be safe. When your active labor has started and your contractions have become more regular, you will definitely need to head into the hospital because the baby is coming.

If, at any time during your third trimester, you start to experience heavy vaginal bleeding or a fever that is higher than 101.5 degrees, or you experience sudden weight gain, pain in the lower stomach, or signs of preterm labor, then you should call your doctor. It is fine to trust your instincts when you experience any symptoms that seem wrong to you.

Things to Do During the Third Trimester

The third trimester is an exciting time. There is so much going on that you need to keep track of. Not only is your baby growing like crazy, but you are also dealing with the different aches and pains that come with this part of pregnancy, and you are preparing your home and your life for the new baby. Some of the things that you can do when you enter the third trimester include:

Keep track of fetal movements. Once you reach 28 weeks, you will want to count the baby's kicks on a regular basis and then note any changes to the activity during that time. This is especially true when you are in the 9th month.

Watch your weight: After you get into the third trimester, your weight gain is going to pick up speed a bit. But it is going to taper down as you get closer to your due date. Some women even report that they lose weight in the end because they eat a healthy diet and the exertion of being pregnant can be hard.

Keep moving. This can be hard now that you have the added weight from the baby, but it is important to keep active as much as possible. For most women, it is just fine to be up and moving as much as possible to help with pregnancy symptoms and to keep you fit. If there is some reason that you should be on bedrest or if there is another issue during this time, your doctor will discuss it with you.

Schedule the checkups for the third trimester. You are going to go through tests like group B strep, anemia, and glucose levels at this time. There will also be an internal examination of your cervix during the final few months to see if you are dilating or effacing at all. The doctor can schedule a nonstress stress if you are a high-risk pregnancy in the final few weeks to make sure that everything is going well.

Take a tour of the hospital. If you didn't do this during your second trimester, then this is the perfect time to do it. Seven months is a great time to look through the birthing center or hospital.

Choose your baby's pediatrician: You should have a few candidates that you want to interview with. Try to meet with them around week 32 and ask them a bunch of questions to see if they are the right one for you.

Buy the baby gear that you need. Make sure that you have all the baby gear that is needed ahead of time. Things like a car seat (the hospital won't let you leave there without having one), stroller, crib, diapers, monitor, and more.

Get educated. A birth class is essential to take in these final weeks. This is very helpful to prepare you more for your entire birth process. You can take birthing classes, take CPR classes, and baby care.

Prepare to breastfeed if you want to do this. There are a lot of benefits to breastfeeding, which is why it is such a great choice for many people. If you choose to breastfeed, you should make sure you are prepared. Take a look at the resources out there to be prepared for breastfeeding and consider getting some of the supplies such as a pump and more.

Learn about the different stages of labor. As you get closer to your due date, the idea of labor may be a scary one for many mothers. But labor is perfectly normal and it is important to know what to expect. Having this information can make it easier to prepare for when the labor actually starts.

Check the birth plan. Talk to your doctor about some of the things that you want to have happened during the birthing process. It is always nice to have a plan in place ahead of time so you make sure that people follow your wishes. But remember that sometimes things change, and you need to be flexible.

Stock up the fridge. One of the best things that you can do for yourself is to make some freezer meals before the baby is born. You are going to spend a lot of time taking care of a baby and recovering after they are born. You don't want to also cook the meals. While some friends and family may drop of meals on occasion, it can be relaxing to know that you have a large supply of healthy meals sitting there and ready to go and that you don't have to cook.

Plan out finances. Your finances are going to change quite a bit when you have a baby. Consider the costs of having a baby and how it is going to affect you financially and come up with a new budget.

Pack your hospital bag. We will discuss this one a bit more soon, but you want to bring along a few necessities, such as clothes to change into, your toothbrush, and more.

Arrange for cord blood banking: If this is something that you have been considering, then this is the time to do it. Make sure that your doctor is aware of these plans so that you get everything that you need. Make sure that you pack any cord blood kit the bank sends with you when you go to the hospital.

The third trimester is an exciting phase for many new mothers. They are excited to meet their new baby, and when they combine this with the aches and pains that come with pregnancy in the third trimester, many are ready for it to be done. Make sure that you get to all of your prenatal appointments and that you follow any recommendations that your doctor gives to you to make sure you finish the pregnancy strong.

Chapter 8:
Getting Ready to Go to the Hospital

As you get to the end of your pregnancy, you are probably getting even more excited about becoming a parent. You want to make sure that everything is as perfect as possible, but you may not know where to start. Here are some ways that you can prepare yourself when you are getting to the end of your pregnancy.

Packing Your Hospital Bag

As you get into the last few weeks of your pregnancy, you will be anxiously awaiting when your baby arrives. One of the things that you might want to consider doing is packing up your hospital bag. You are going to spend a few days in the hospital; about one to three for mothers of vaginal deliveries and three to five days for c-sections, as long as everything goes well. You don't want to end up at the hospital without something that is important or something that you need during that time. Working on your hospital bag can make it easier to be comfortable while you stay in the hospital with your baby.

Each woman is going to be a bit different in what they want to bring to the hospital with them. You can always pick out what you think is the best for your needs. Make sure that you bring along some of your necessities, such as your toothbrush and toothpaste, deodorant, and shower supplies. Some of the other things that you may want to consider putting into the bag include:

- *A dressing gown*: If you plan to walk up and down the halls during early labor, this can be helpful. Since many hospitals are warm, you may want to pick out one that is lightweight. Go with a darker color or one that is busy to help hide stains during this time.

- *Slippers*: Pick ones that are backless so that you can get them on and off easier.

- *Socks*: Sometimes, women complain of feet that are cold during labor.

- *Lotion or massage oil*: This can be useful if you want to be massaged during the labor.

- *Lip balm*: In a warm labor ward, it is likely that your lips will dry out fast. Bring some lip balm to avoid discomfort.

- *Snack and drinks*: These can be nice for something to eat after labor. Some hospitals will allow you to have snacks during labor but check ahead of time.

- *Things to pass the time or help you relax*: These can be nice during labor because they help you to focus on something other than the actual labor. They can also be nice while you are in the hospital healing. Some things that you can bring along include music, a computer, magazines, and books.

- *A going home outfit*: You will want to have some comfortable clothes that are a little loose to wear in the hospital and on the way home. You can also bring a home outfit for the baby to come home in.

- *Baby car seat.* Hospitals in the United States won't let you head home without a car seat so make sure you have it there with you.

- *Nursing bras.* It is best to bring at least a few of these with you.

- *Diapers.* The hospital may provide a few of these, but bring some just in case.

Your chosen baby blankets. Many babies like to cuddle with a blanket and their moms, and if it is cold outside when you leave the hospital, you will be glad you have this.

- Breast pads

- Maternity pads

- A few sleepsuits or other outfits that you want the baby to wear.

- Hot, socks, and booties.

These are just a few of the things that you may want to consider adding to your hospital bag. Get this prepared a few weeks ahead of time in case labor starts before your 40 weeks are done. Then you can just grab the bag and head out the door, knowing that everything you will need is right there with you.

Writing Your Birthing Plan

One thing that a lot of expectant mothers like to focus on is writing out a birth plan. This is definitely something that you should discuss with your doctor, perhaps during the second trimester, to see how many of your requests are reasonable and that the doctor will try to accommodate. This gives many women a sense of power over the situation and can make it easier on the mother heading into the experience.

The first step is to get out a journal and write down as many plans and thoughts that come to your head about the upcoming birth. This journal is going to be used to help you establish what is a priority and can give you a list of thoughts that will make the birth plan easier to create.

Your birth plan is a simple statement, one that is usually about one page, that talks about the preferences that you would like to see during the birth of your child. You can then provide a copy of this to everyone who will be in contact with you during the delivery.

Now, this is not a way to go through and write out a big list of demands to the doctor and the medical staff. It is simply a way to make sure that the doctors are aware of what you would like. Many mothers may say they want to do an all-natural birth, with no medications. Some may request that they get to have time with skin to skin contact with their baby before any tests are done. It is not acceptable to have a birthing plan that is twenty pages long though.

Also, it is important to remain as flexible as possible about the desires you have, because there are many times when things don't go according to your plan. Yes, you may wish to have a natural birth without any interventions, but when the baby goes into distress, your doctor may need to do an emergency c-section. The birthing plan can be a great way to ensure others know your preferences, but remember that childbirth is not always predictable and your birthing plan may not get followed exactly.

Picking Out Birthing Classes

There are many types of birthing classes that you can consider. Each one is going to be a bit different, and the one you go with may have to do with your birthing plan or how you want to do your birth experience. Many hospitals offer up a general birthing class that can give you a lot of the basics. But there are also several methods that you can consider, and which can be helpful during labor as well. Let's take a look at some of these options and see which one you like the best.

The Lamaze Technique

This is the first type of child birthing class you may want to consider. Lamaze is one of the most widely used methods that are used in the United States because the approach that it gives mothers to childbirth is healthy and natural. Lamaze doesn't discourage or support the use of medical interventions or other medicines that can be used during your labor and delivery, which is part of why it is so popular to use. Instead, it is there to inform mothers about all of their options so they can make the right decision for themselves, rather than being pushed one way or the other.

One of the main focuses of Lamaze is to help build up your confidence about childbirth and helping you to keep the birth of your baby as safe and simple as possible. There are often breathing techniques that are taught as well which can help you through the pain of contractions, whether you are using medicine or not with your experience.

The classes for Lamaze are usually pretty small and will be a minimum of 12 hours. These classes often touch on topics such as:

* Healthy lifestyle choices both during and after birth

- Breastfeeding

- Medical procedures

- Effective skills to use with a communication

- Getting the right support during labor

- How to practice staying relaxed during labor by using internal and external focus points.

- The best breathing techniques that you can use during labor.

- Relaxation techniques and even massage that can be used during the birth.

- Different ways that you can try to position yourself when you are going through birth and labor to make things easier.

- Normal labor, birth, and postpartum care.

The Bradley Method

This method is known as the husband coached birth. It is a method that will help a mother deliver without the use of pain medications and can prepare the father of the baby to be the birch coach of the mom. Although this method is mostly meant to help prepare a mother to give birth without any medications, it could also help you be prepared for any situations that come up and that you are not expecting, such as needing an emergency c-section.

This is a course that will take place over twelve sessions. In these sessions, you will learn:

- How important exercise and nutrition are during pregnancy

- Some different relaxation techniques that you can do for pain management

- Practicing for labor.

- How to avoid a c-section birth unless necessary.

- Postpartum care of the mother

- Breastfeeding

- Guidance for a coach for how to support the mother.

The Alexander Technique

This is a technique that is meant to improve the ease and freedom of coordination, flexibility, balance, and movement. You will ideally try to take these lessons each week while you are pregnant because it is more of an education process. The more that you practice this, the greater the benefits. Although this is a technique that can be useful for everyone, the goals for mothers who try this method are:

- To ease some of the discomforts that can come from nursing.

- Aid in recovering after giving birth

- An increase in how effective they are at pushing during the delivery

- An improved level of comfort during the pregnancy

Hypnobirthing

This is known as a Mangan method. This is a relaxed and natural childbirth education approach. This method is going to teach the mother how to use some self-hypnosis techniques to make it easier to handle labor. Teachers are going to spend time emphasizing childbirth and pregnancy, as well as on pre-birth parenting. This series is going to be five classes that are about two and a half hours long each.

These are just a few of the different child birthing classes that you can consider using. Each mother is different and you need to pick out the method that works the best for you.

Consider Baby CPR

You may want to consider doing a class that has information on baby CPR. You never know when your little one may get something stuck in their mouth or have trouble with breathing. Being certified in baby CPR can help give you the peace of mind of knowing that your baby will be safe at all times.

Permanent damage to the brain and even death could occur if the baby isn't able to breathe and blood flow stops. This is why every parent who is in charge of taking care of their child or an infant should know how to do this kind of CPR. There are classes in most areas, so looking at the website www.heart.org to find out where the classes are to you.

Many times, one of the other birthing classes that you pick will include some of these baby CPR classes as well. See if this is true for yours. If not, consider taking some time to become certified to make sure that you can always take care of your baby, even if the worst happens.

Do I Want to Do Cord Blood Banking?

Another thing that you may want to consider when you are getting ready for the hospital is to decide whether you want to do cord blood banking. Cord blood is the blood that is going to stay on the umbilical cord and the placenta after the birth. Most births discard this blood. However, you can use cord blood banking to help store and preserve the cord blood from your baby. If you are looking to do this, you must make sure that you work with a blood bank that is accredited by the AABB, or American Association of Blood Banks.

The cord blood is an important source of stem cells, ones that are specifically related through genetics to your baby and the rest of your family. These stem cells are considered dominant in the way that they can help systems, organs, and tissues develop in the body.

Stem cells are able to help transform some of the other cell types in the body in order to get them to create new growth and development. They are also important parts of the immune system. The transformation of these stem cells will help provide doctors with a way to treat some health disorders that are inherited and even treat leukemia.

The stem cells from this cord blood could be effective. Not only could it help with treating certain conditions for the baby, but also for siblings and parents. These blood stem cells have a similar ability to help treat the disease as bone marrow currently does, but there is actually less risk from rejection. Basically, this is a type of insurance against future disease, either in your baby or in someone else in your family. Hopefully, you would never run into a medical situation that would need these stem cells. But it can bring some peace of mind knowing that this resource is available if it is needed.

Once the cord blood is collected after the baby is born (make sure your doctor knows you want to do this so they don't discard the blood before you can get it), the blood is going to be processed before being stored in a laboratory facility, known as a blood bank. You can choose the blood bank you want to use, just make sure they have the right accreditation.

The collection of the cord blood has no indication of health risk which is good news. Since the retrieval is done after the cord has been cut, there shouldn't be any harm, discomfort, or pain. This helps to make the process as safe as possible.

The costs that you incur when you do this will depend on the bank that you choose to go with. There are often two fees that are involved in this kind of banking. The first is going to be the initial fee that will cover your enrollment, the collection, and then the storage for about the first year of this process. The second is going to be the storage fee that you pay for each year.

Depending on how much storage time is included in the initial amount, the fee that you pay in the beginning will range from $900 to $2100. Annual storage fees, after this time, will be about $100. It is common for many storage facilities to offer some prepaid plants at a discount, and some payment plans, so that you are more willing to store with them.

Deciding to do cord blood banking is a completely personal choice. Some parents know that they have a family history of some illnesses and diseases, so they choose to do this kind of treatment. Others decide they want to do it for peace of mind. It is a good idea to have a discussion about this before the birth to determine what you want to do.

Chapter 9:
Getting Ready for Labor: Stages of Labor

Your child's birth, whether it is your first child or your fourth, is a special experience. All deliveries are different and unique and there's no telling how yours will go. But no matter what, there are stages of each labor process, and knowing about them and what to expect can make a big difference in how you prepare.

Childbirth is going to occur through three stages. The first stage is the time when true labor starts. It continues going until the cervix has dilated all the way to 10 centimeters. The second stage is going to be the period of time after the cervix has dilated to the ten centimeters until the baby is delivered and in your arms. And the third stage is when the placenta is delivered. Let's take a look at each stage of labor and explore what happens in each one.

The First Stage of Labor
The longest stage of your labor is the first stage. This is pretty much every-thing that happens from the first real labor contraction that you feel all the way until you are ready to start pushing the baby out. It will have three phases that occur during it including:

- Early labor: This is the time when the first contraction occurs until the cervix reaches 3 centimeters.

- Active labor phase: This is going to be the phase that goes from three centimeters until the cervix reaches seven centimeters.

- Transition phase: This goes all the way until the cervix reaches full dilation.

Each phase is different and distinct. And the mother is going to find that there are different challenges, both physical and emotional, that they will deal with.

Early Labor Phase

During this phase, it is important to relax as much as possible. While the contractions may be painful and hard, this stage doesn't need to send you to the hospital or to your birthing center. Try to stay home and enjoy the comfort of your familiar surroundings, rather than getting straight to the hospital. If your early labor does occur during the day, try to lay back and take it easy, or even do a few simple routines in the house if you can.

The goal here is to keep yourself occupied while still conserving your energy as much as possible. For some women, this phase can progress quickly. But it is also possible for you to stay in this type of labor for many hours. The contractions are noticeable and may cause some pain, but you should still be able to move around and talk and do some regular activities.

During this time, make sure to eat some small snacks and drink water so that you can keep your energy up. Keep track of your contractions and time them so you have a basis point to refer to later when they get worse. If it is night time, and you are able to, try to get some sleep to help with your energy levels. If you can't fall asleep (and it is fine if you can't) concentrate on doing some small activities, such as packing your bag, doing a few dishes, or something else to distract yourself.

Some of the things that you can expect when you are in this early phase of labor include:

This type of labor will last about eight to twelve hours. This amount can change. Some women may get through this phase in a few hours though, so listen to your body and see if the contractions are getting worse. But until that happens, it is fine to sit back and relax or do some light chores around the house.

- During this phase, your cervix is going to efface and dilate out to three centimeters.

- Your contractions will usually last between thirty to 45 seconds each, and you will get somewhere between five to thirty minutes in between them.

- The contractions that you feel are usually going to be mild and, in the beginning, they will be irregular. But they will get stronger and more frequent as the labor progresses.

Contractions can feel different for everyone. Sometimes, they will feel like menstrual cramps. Sometimes, they will be a pain in your lower back, and sometimes, they will be a tightening or a pressure in the area of the pelvis.

Amniotic sac rupture may happen during this first stage of labor wherein your water breaks. Some people notice that their water breaks right at the beginning, but it isn't uncommon for it to break much later on when you are at the hospital.

When you are experiencing contractions, you need to pay attention to them. Notice if they are growing more intense as time goes on, if they are lasting longer or getting closer together, or if they seem to be following a regular pattern at all. And if the water does break, notice the odor and the color of the fluid. Also, keep track of the time it breaks because if too much time passes between the water breaking and the baby being born, it can increase the risk for infections.

If you have a support person around, whether it is a family member your spouse, or someone like a doula, there are a few things that they can do to help out as well. These include:

- The support person should keep up their strength as well. They need to be there to help the delivery and this requires energy as well.

- The support person can suggest some simple activities that can help to draw the focus of the mom away from the labor.

- The support person can offer support, reassurance, and comfort to mom.

- The support person should try to be a calming influence to the mom.

Work on timing the contractions. The mom is probably not going to remember to time these contractions, but that is important to the process. The support person can help with that.

Active Labor Phase

When you reach the active labor phase, it is time to head into the birth center or to the hospital. Your contractions during this stage are going to be longer, stronger, and much closer together. If possible, you will need to surround yourself with a lot of support. This is also the time when you will want to start some of the breathing techniques, and the relaxation exercises, between your contractions.

While you are at the hospital, you will want to make sure that you can switch your positions often during this phase. This can make the contractions easier to manage and can ensure that the labor goes faster. You can try to take a warm bath, try sitting in a different position, and even walking to help. Continue to drink plenty of water during this phase if the hospital allows it.

- There are a few things that you can expect during this phase. These things include:

- Your active labor is going to last about three to five hours.

- During this time, the cervix is going to dilate from four to seven centimeters.

- The contractions are going to get longer and closer. They will usually last between 45 to 60 seconds with up to five minutes of rest in between them.

- The contractions are going to feel a lot stronger.

- You can consider calling your doctor to make sure, but this is usually the time to head into the hospital.

Transition Labor Phase

The support person will most likely be relied on heavily by the mother during this phase. This phase is very challenging to get through, even though it is the shortest of the three. As the mother, try to use your breathing exercises and remember that you only have to get through one contraction at a time. If the contractions are close together, this is sometimes hard to do. But remember how far you have already come. When you start to feel the urge to push, it is time to get the baby out, and you should tell your healthcare provider right away.

This is a fast-paced phase of labor, and it is the last one before the baby is born. There are a few things that you can expect from this phase including:

- This phase is going to last somewhere between half an hour to two hours.

- Your cervix is going to dilate from 8 to 10 centimeters.

- The contractions during this phase are going to increase. They will usually last between 60 to 90 seconds, and there will be somewhere between a 30 second to 2-minute rest between each one.

- At this time, the contractions are going to be intense, strong, and long. And depending on how far along you are in this stage, they can even overlap.

- It is most often the hardest phase; however, the good news is that it can be the shortest.

- Each woman is different, but you may also experience side effects such as gas, vomiting, nausea, chills, or hot flashes during this time.

The Second Stage of Pregnancy

Once you go through the first stage of labor and have been dealing with the contractions for some time, it is time to move on to the second stage of labor. This is the time when you feel your body automatically trying to push the baby out, even without your help, and the doctor has said you are at ten centimeters. The second stage is going to involve all the pushing and then the delivery of the baby. Up to this point, the hormones in the body have made it possible to get to this point. But now you are going to have to step up and help out a little with pushing.

What Can I Expect When Pushing?

Many women who haven't gone through labor before may be curious what the pushing phase is like. Some of the things that you can expect during this phase of labor include:

- The pushing phase can expect anywhere from twenty minutes to two hours.

- The contractions are going to last between 45 to 90 seconds with three to five minutes in between.

- You will feel a strong natural urge to push. Pushing when you feel that urge can really help to expedite the process.

- You may feel a strong pressure at the rectum and some women will have a urination or minor bowel accident because of the pressure.

- After some time of pushing, the head of the baby is going to crown or become visible.

- You may feel a burning or stinging sensation during this crowning process, but each woman is different.

- During the crowning, your doctor is going to ask you not to push. Try to resist the urge to push here.

Try to find a position where you can have an advantage using gravity when you are pushing. Then, just push when you feel the urge. When you are in between the contractions, try to rest as much as possible to help get back some of your strength, or at least preserve it a little bit. If you want to, it is sometimes recommended to use a mirror so you can view your progress and get some encouragement when you see how far you have come. When it is time to push, don't hold back and use as much energy as you can to push.

One neat thing to know is that when you are in labor, your child is actually getting himself prepares to enter the outside world. They are an active participant and as long as everything goes well, they will also take steps to make sure that they can enter the world correctly. Some of the things that you will see your baby doing during this phase include:

- The head of the baby is going to turn over to one side and then the chin is going to rest on the chest automatically. This allows the back of the head to lead the way, which makes things easier.

- Once your body has had time to dilate fully, the head of the baby is going to lead the way. Then the torso and the head will begin to turn towards your back as they get down to the vagina.

- From here, the baby's head will start to emerge or crown through your vaginal opening.

- Once the baby's head is out, then the head and shoulders will turn to face your side to make it easier for the baby just to slip out.

What to Expect with Delivery?

Some women are not sure what to expect when they give birth for the first time. One thing to keep in mind is that when you do deliver, your baby has been soaking in the placenta, and in amniotic fluid, for the past nine months. Following all your contractions and a passage through your narrow birth canal, there may be some characteristics of the baby that are perfectly normal, but which you were not prepared for. Some of these include:

- Enlarged genitals

- Lanugo. This is a fine downy hair that is going to cover up the temple, forehead, back, and shoulders of the baby.

- Puffy eyes

- A vernix coating: This is a cheese-looking substance that can coat the fetus in the uterus.

- A head that is cone shaped.

The Third Stage of Labor: Delivering the Placenta

After the birth of your child, there is actually another stage of labor to go through. This third stage is the placenta's delivery. It is the stage where you will deliver the shortest and will only spend five to thirty minutes in total.

After your baby is delivered, your health care provider is going to be watching to see if there are any small contractions that occur with you again. These contractions signal that the placenta is separating from the uterine wall and that it is ready to be delivered.

It is also possible that a massage is done to apply pressure or the umbilical cord be gently pulled by the healthcare professionals. This results in the delivery of your placenta. Some mothers experience severe shivering and shaking after this happens, and this is completely normal and not something to be concerned about.

For the next few hours you may be monitored after you complete all of these stages of childbirth. This is to make sure that your uterus keeps contracting to heal and that the bleeding doesn't become excessive.

What Happens During A C-Section?

The birth that we described above is for a vaginal delivery. It can be done with or without medication to help the mother get through the pain. But there are times when you will need to have a c-section. Sometimes these are planned, such as when the mother has a complication when the baby needs to be delivered early, when the baby is in distress during labor, or when the mother is carrying more than one baby. Understanding what to expect during a pregnancy, whether it is a planned c-section or not, can make a difference in how you recover after the c-section is done.

With a c-section, your doctor is going to start out by explaining why they think it is necessary to perform cesarean section. A form of consent will be required to be signed by you. An obstetrician/midwife that can do the surgery will be assigned to you.

In most cases, your partner or husband can be with you during the preparation and during the birth. Sometimes the c-section, will be an emergency and there won't be time for your partner to change, they may not be allowed to stay in the operating room with you.

The anesthesiologist will then come in, if it is not an emergency, to review some of the pain management options that you can go with. It is never very common to be given general anesthesia anymore, except in an extreme situation. Usually, you are just given something for regional pain relief, like a spinal block or epidural. This helps you to have your lower half numb, but you will still be alert for when your baby is born.

If you had an epidural to help with pain relief during labor, you will also use the same pain relief during your cesarean section. Before the surgery, the doctor will give you some extra medication to ensure that you won't feel much during the surgery. Sometimes, you will feel a bit of tugging during the surgery, but there shouldn't be any pain. In this procedure, the urine is drained out from the urethra using a catheter. They will start the IV next to help with fluids and medications. You will then be moved over to the operating room.

During the procedure, you will be given antibiotics as well to help prevent any infections after the operation. The doctors will then administer the anesthesia and raise a screen so you won't see the surgery they make. You can choose to see the baby if you would like, just ask the nurse to lower the screen to see the baby.

Once your anesthesia has taken effect, the belly is going to have some antiseptic put on it. The doctor is then going to make a small horizontal incision above your pubic bone. They will then cut through all the underlying tissue, working their way down to the uterus. When the doctor reaches the abdominal muscles, they will manually separate them and spread apart to show the uterus underneath. The doctor can then reach in and pull out the baby. Once they have time to cut the cord, you will have a moment to see the baby before they hand them off to the nurse or the pediatrician. While the staff takes some time to examine the baby, the doctor is going to deliver the placenta and will then close up the incisions they made.

After taking some time to examine the baby, the nurse will hand them to your partner, who then has the option to hold them next to you. You can nuzzle, kiss, and talk to your baby while the doctor finishes stitching you up.

Over time, the stitches that are used to close up the incision will dissolve. The final layer may be closed up with staples or stitches, which will be removed three to seven days later. Sometimes, the doctor will use stitches that can dissolve. After the surgery is done, you will be moved over to the recovery room where you will be watched for the next few hours. If the baby is doing fine, they will be in the room with you and you can hold them. You will have to keep the IV in to help with eating and drinking.

At this time, if you plan to breastfeed, then this is the time to do it. You may find that nursing is the most comfortable for you and for the baby if you lie on your sides facing each other. Those who have c-sections are going to stay in the hospital for three days unless there are other complications. Your doctor will discuss your pain medication with you and how to treat your surgery after you go home.

Many mothers may not be prepared for a c-section. This can really change up their birthing plans, and they may be confused as to what is going on. C-sections are generally safe, especially if the baby made it to full term. You will just need to spend more time recovering. Most women who have c-sections will need to take about six weeks before they are feeling better and able to do the regular exercise again.

Heidi Oster

Chapter 10:
In-Hospital Procedures Commonly Done on a Newborn

After your baby is born, you may be curious about what is going to happen now. Many practitioners are going to allow you to hold onto the baby right after they are born. Warm towels or some blankets will be placed over you and the baby in order to make sure that the baby is warm. This is an important time for bonding and many birth centers and hospitals will give you that time before they do any other tests. Then, when you or the baby are both ready, there are some tests that all hospitals will go through.

This newborn testing is very important and it is something that you should think about before the birth. During pregnancy, we are going to focus so much on the actual birth that sometimes we may not even think about this newborn testing. There are several different tests that will be done at your hospital, and some of the most common ones include:

Measuring the Length and Weight
The timing of these tests can vary based on your hospital, but they will be done at some point during the first few hours of your baby's life. Some hospitals will do it after a few minutes of skin-to-skin contact, and others will wait. Most professionals believe that this is a bad thing because the bonding period is so important. The baby only has a short amount of time when they

are alert after birth and many professionals believe they should use this time to bond with the parents.

Many parents are now writing out their birth plans so that the procedures for these tests are put off until later. They usually try to delay this for the first hour or so after the baby is born. You can talk to your doctor to see what their rules are for your hospital and if there is any room to move the timing of this.

Doing Eye Drops

Eye drops have changed in many states recently. In the past, Silver Nitrate was used in most hospitals. This would burn the baby's eyes a bit, but it was used to help prevent an infection. It is now becoming more common for hospitals to use erythromycin instead. Make sure that you talk to your doctor to see which one is being used.

While the eye drops are important to help prevent infections in the baby, it is still another thing that you can delay until later on. Most states say that it is up to your doctor to put the eye drops in, but there isn't a time indicated there. This means that you and your doctor can decide when to put these drops in. As long as you get these done in the first few hours, it will be fine.

A Vitamin K Injection

This is another injection that the baby will need to get after birth. Babies are not going to be born with a good clotting system. This is where the vitamin K injection came into place. This became law when force deliveries were common in order to prevent any bleeding in the brain due to trauma that this procedure could cause to the head.

Today, it is still common to give the vitamin K injection, despite the fact that most deliveries are not done with the forceps any longer. This is because vitamin K can provide some good benefits to the baby. Some countries have different policies on when to provide this injection rather than doing it all of the time. This injection is something that you should consider talking with your doctor to figure out what will work the best for you.

Newborn Screening and PKU Testing

Newborn screening is a term that is used to define the whole set of tests that is done in order to screen your baby for a variety of diseases, including PKU. While many moms state that they are having this PKU screening, it is common that the newborn screening is going to be done for many disorders all at the same time. The tests that are done will vary depending on the state.

The newborn screening is going to involve sticking the foot of your baby for blood. This test is only going to be accurate when the baby has received a diet that contains phenylalanine, which can come from artificial formulas and milk, for at least 24 hours. This is why a baby is breastfed until at least one day after they are born. Taking it earlier than this could give you results that are not accurate.

Hepatitis Vaccine Administration

This is now a vaccine that most states will require you to have. You will have two choices for when you can start this vaccine though. You can either give it to your child when they are first born, or you can do it when you have their two-month check-up. You should first look at your own risk for developing hepatitis and then decide on the best time to give it to your child.

Apgar Testing

This test is technically the first test that your baby will get. In most places, it is done in the first few moments that the baby is born before they even hand the baby over to you. Often, the parents don't know that it happened. This test is simply an evaluation of the way that the baby sounds and looks when they are first born.

The medical professional is going to give a score for each sign at one minute and at five minutes after birth. If there seem to be any issues with the baby, an additional score can be given at ten minutes. A score that is between seven and ten is normal, four to seven might need some help from the doctor, and if the score is at three or below, it means that the baby needs immediate medical attention.

Remember, this score does not correspond with the intelligence levels, or the SAT score, that your child will have later in life. In some circles, this test is seen as not very useful. For example, a baby who needs help or who is in distress is not going to wait or be left alone until the doctor performs the APGAR at one minute. This is a harmless test, but many doctors are going to choose other methods to help watch the baby.

Depending on the type of pregnancy you had and how the baby is doing, there may be other tests that your doctor will want to perform. They may want to do blood sugar testing, hearing tests, and more. Make sure to talk to your doctor about the tests that they wish to complete so you are fully informed about what will happen after delivery.

Chapter 11:
Post Recovery

After your baby is born, there is a lot that you need to keep track of. During this time, you are getting used to your changing body, to the new baby, and even to some physical pains. If you had a c-section, the time can take even longer before you feel better. As a new mother, you need to take some special care of your body after giving birth, and while breastfeeding as well. Doing this will help you to regain your energy and your strength. Let's take a look at some of the steps that you can take to help recover from birth.

Getting Your Rest
After you have been released from the hospital (one to three days for vaginal delivery and three to five days for a c-section as long as there aren't any complications), you should spend the first few days relaxing as much as possible. You need to focus your energy on yourself and spend this time getting familiar with your baby.

Even though there are probably a ton of excited requests from family and friends to come over and meet the baby, try to limit your visitors so that you can get as much rest as you can. Do not put a lot of unnecessary expectations on yourself. For example, you do not need to keep your house sparkling clean. During that first bit of time at home, you may only be able to sleep, eat, and take care of your baby, and there is nothing wrong with that. Try to lie down and sleep when the baby sleeps. Don't worry about cleaning the house. And if others offer, allow them to help out when they can.

Physical Changes

After your baby is born, your doctor will spend some time talking to you about some of the changes that you will go through as your body works at recovering. Some of the things you may notice include:

- There may be some swelling in the feet and legs. The best way to deal with this is to keep your feet elevated when you can.

- There is the possibility that you will feel constipated. Some fresh produce and plenty of water can help with this.

It is common to feel some menstrual like cramping, especially for those who are breastfeeding. Your milk will come in sometime between three and six weeks after delivery. Even if you are not breastfeeding, you may have some milk leaking and your breasts could feel uncomfortable, full, or tender.

Follow the instructions your doctor gives for how much activity such as walking, doing chores, and more, that you are allowed to do.

During your postpartum visit, which occurs about six weeks after birth, your doctor will check in on your recovery. You can take that time to ask about resuming some of your normal activities. Ask about the right fitness and eating plans to help you get back to a healthy weight over time.

You should also take this time to talk about sex and birth control with your doctor unless you would like to have two kids right on top of each other. It is possible that your period would return within six to eight weeks, or even sooner if you don't breastfeed. For some women who breastfeed, your period may not come back for many months. The best way to prevent a pregnancy until you are ready is to find a reliable form of birth control.

Regaining A Healthy Weight

Both the pregnancy and the labor you go through at the end will have an effect on your body. After you give birth, it is likely that you will lose around ten pounds right away because of the weight of the baby, the placenta, and the fluids that you lost as well. It is not a good idea to try and lose any additional pregnancy weight right away. Slow weight loss over several months is the best method, especially if you plan to breastfeed. Mothers who are nursing can safely lose a moderate amount of weight without any worries about how their milk supply will be influenced.

A healthy eating plan and some regular exercise might be enough for some women to return to their healthy weight. If you find that you aren't really losing weight, or it is taking too long, make sure that you cut back on foods that have extra sugars and fats, soft drinks, desserts, and so on. When you focus your energy on a well-balanced diet, you can help yourself lose weight while also giving yourself and your baby the nutrition you need.

Feeling Blue

After you give birth, it is normal to feel sad, weepy, and overwhelmed for a few days. This is pretty common due to the changing hormones, some anxiety about how to care for the baby, and a general lack of sleep because you have a newborn. All of these are normal, and it is important to be patient with yourself here. They will usually go away quickly. But if you notice that your sadness is lasting more than two weeks, you should go see your doctor. Even if it is before your postpartum visit, go ahead and do this.

You could be dealing with a serious, but very treatable condition known as postpartum depression. It is possible that postpartum depression can happen at any time within your first year after giving birth. Some of the signs that you will notice with postpartum depression include:

- Thoughts about harming either yourself or your baby

- Having no interest or not getting any pleasure from various activities such as socializing or sex.

- Feeling guilty or worthless

- Not having much interest in your baby

- Being worried all the time about the baby

- Trouble with focusing, remembering things, or making any decisions

- Overeating and weight gain

- Not being able to eat and then losing weight

- Having trouble with sleeping, being tired, or a combination of both.

- Having chest pains, headaches, heart palpitations, hyperventilation or numbness

- No energy at all.

- Crying often, feeling depressed or sad.

- Feeling irritable or restless.

Some women are not going to talk about the symptoms they are feeling because they may feel guilty or embarrassed about them. Don't let this happen to you. This kind of depression can make it hard for some women to take care of their baby, and it could lead to issues with emotional bonding and developmental milestones in your baby. Your doctor can help you to feel better and can get you back to enjoying the baby. Medicine and or therapy can help to treat this kind of depression.

Chapter 12:
FAQ's

What Is the Best Sleeping Position When You Are Pregnant?

The best position to sleep in is one that will keep the curve of your back in line. Sleeping on your side with one of the knees bent can work nicely. Just make sure that you aren't lying with the knees all the way up to your chest. During the third trimester, it is best to avoid lying on your back because it will make the heart work more and can cause a big backache. Lying on your stomach during this time may not be comfortable and it can add pressure to the fetus. Use a pillow under the head, but not on your shoulders. Some women find that having a pillow between their legs can help as well.

What Are Some of The Early Symptoms of Pregnancy?

Outside of a missed period, there are some other symptoms that you may notice when you are pregnant. Pregnancy can bring about changes in your hormonal balance, and this could include a variety of symptoms like:

- Frequent urination

- Constipation

- Mood swings

- Headaches

- Fainting and dizziness

Why Do I Have So Many Cravings When I Am Pregnant?

Some women will find that they have strong cravings, or they can't stand certain foods once they become pregnant. This is related to all the hormonal changes that occur during this time. This effect is often so strong that some women will find that their stomachs just can't stand some of the foods that used to be their favorites.

How Long Do the Cravings and Nausea Last During Pregnancy?

It is possible for some women that the food aversions, cravings, and nausea will last for your whole pregnancy. But for most women, these symptoms are going to lessen between the 13th and 14th week of the pregnancy. Until that happens, it is important to eat a diet that is as healthy as possible to ensure that your baby can get the essential nutrients they need. If you are having trouble eating because of nausea, then it is important to talk to your doctor about this.

What Nutrients Should I Look for Inside My Prenatal Vitamins?

Some of the nutrients, and their amounts, that you should aim for in your prenatal vitamin include:

- 150 micrograms of iodine

- 17 mg iron

- 15 mg zinc

- 10 mg vitamin E

- 6 mcg vitamin B12

- 20 mg niacin

- 2 mg riboflavin

- 3 mg thiamine

- 70 mg vitamin C

- 200 or more mg calcium

- 400 IU vitamin D

- 400 mcg folic acid

What Is the Difference Between Effaced and Dilated?

Effaced means how thinned out the cervix is and dilated is how opened up it is. You need to have the cervix effaced to 100 percent and then it needs to be dilated to 10 centimeters before you are able to deliver your baby.

What Are the Benefits of Breastfeeding My Baby?

There are a number of benefits your baby can enjoy when you breastfeed, and it is even beneficial to mom too! Some of the benefits of breastfeeding your baby includes:

- It can provide some antibodies that will help your baby resist illness

- It is easier to digest compared to formula. This means the baby will be less gassy and constipated.

- It can help to reduce the risk of SIDS in your baby.

- Some studies find that babies who were breastfed may have higher levels of cognitive function.

- Breast milk may be able to help your baby fight against lymphoma, leukemia, high cholesterol, and diabetes.

Do I Need to Make Changes in My Diet If I Have Diabetes?

If you find out you have diabetes during your pregnancy, or you had diabetes as a pre-existing condition before your pregnancy, then you may need to work with your doctor to adjust your diet. Changing your diabetes diet while you are pregnant can help you avoid some issues with high or low blood sugar levels.

How Does My Doctor Figure Out When My Pregnancy Started?

Most of the time, it is hard to know the exact day that you got pregnant. The doctor will usually count your pregnancy start from the first day of the last menstrual period. This is often about two weeks ahead of when conception occurred.

Are Prescription Drugs Harmful to My Baby While I'm Pregnant

Some medications can be harmful to the baby when you are pregnant. If you are on any medications, you should talk to your doctor about those medications and if they are still safe to take while you are pregnant. If you develop an issue during the pregnancy, your doctor will decide if a prescription medication is the best option for you, or if you should go with something else.

Why Would I Need to Have My Labor Induced?

There are several reasons why your doctor may decide to induce your pregnancy. Some of these include:

- You are past your due date by one or two weeks. The longer you go past your due date, the higher the risk you will have for complications.

- Your water breaks, but labor doesn't start. Once the water breaks, you and the baby could get an infection.

- You have some other health problem that could put the baby at risk. Issues like preeclampsia, high blood pressure, and diabetes could make it so you will want to induce water.

- A test that your doctor did may show that the baby has a problem. If the baby isn't growing right or they have an abnormal heart rate, the doctor may decide to induce you.

What Happens During My Oral Glucose Tolerance Test?

This test is going to involve the mother quickly drinking a special sweetened liquid. This drink has about 50g of glucose. The body is able to absorb this glucose quickly, which can cause your levels of blood glucose to rise within an hour. Then you will give a blood sample to measure how the glucose was stored by the body. It can help indicate if you have gestational diabetes.

Can I Exercise While I Am Pregnant?

Yes, it is fine to exercise while you are pregnant. In most cases, it is fine to exercise at the levels that you did before your pregnancy. Just make sure you are comfortable and that you have approval from your doctor.

What Are Some of The Advantages of Genetic Testing?

One benefit of doing genetic testing is to find out any problems that may be unknown before this. Many flawed genes that these tests are able to find won't be linked to your family history, ethnicity, or race. You may not have known that you or your partner carry these issues and knowing the risk can help you make some better decisions about your family.

These tests can also provide you with some answers about your family history. The results have shown many families if they are in a high-risk group. The test is easy to do because you simply take a saliva or blood sample before you are pregnant and it is harmless and quick to do.

What Are Braxton Hicks Contractions?

Many women are going to have a harmless false labor pain known as Braxton Hicks contractions. These are pretty erratic, and they are not going to get closer together. They often stop when you either rest or move around. These are not considered a part of the level. If you are not sure about which types of contractions you are dealing with, then you should get medical help.

Conclusion

Thank you for making it through to the end of *What to Expect for First Time Moms*. Let's hope it was informative and able to provide you with all of the tools you need to achieve your goals whatever they may be.

The next step is to use this guidebook to help you get through the different parts of your pregnancy. Pregnancy is an exciting time, but many new expectant mothers aren't sure about what is going to happen at each stage of their pregnancy. This guidebook is meant to provide you with the information that you need, whether you want to know how to pick out a doctor, what happens during each week of the pregnancy, or even what to expect during labor and beyond.

If you find this book helpful in anyway a review to support my endeavors is much appreciated.

Lightning Source UK Ltd.
Milton Keynes UK
UKHW021019080822
407000UK00009B/277